THE POCKET

ESSENTIAL OILS

Published in 2025
by Gemini Books
Part of Gemini Books Group

Based in Woodbridge and London

Marine House, Tide Mill Way,
Woodbridge, Suffolk IP12 1AP
United Kingdom

www.geminibooks.com

Cover image: Shutterstock Ltd/New Africa

ISBN 978-1-80247-296-7

A CIP catalogue record for this book is available from the British Library.

Manufacturer's EU Representative: Eurolink Compliance Limited, 25 Herbert
Place, Dublin, D02 AY86, Republic of Ireland. admin@eurolink-europe.ie.

Disclaimer: This book is intended for general informational purposes only
and should not be relied upon as recommending or promoting any specific
practice or method of health treatments. It is not intended to diagnose,
treat or prevent any illness or condition and is not a substitute for advice
from a health care professional. You should consult your health practitioner
before engaging in any of informational detailed in this book. You should
not use the information in this book as a substitute for health or other
treatment prescribed by a professional practitioner. The publisher makes no
representations or warranties with respect to the accuracy, completeness
or currency of the contents of this work, and specifically disclaim, without
limitation, any implied warranties of merchantability or fitness for
a particular purpose and any injury, illness, damage, liability or loss incurred,
directly or indirectly, from the use or application of any of the contents of this
book. Furthermore, the publisher is not affiliated with and does not sponsor or
endorse any methods of treatment or products referred in this book.

Printed in China

10 9 8 7 6 5 4 3 2 1

FSC
MIX
Paper | Supporting
responsible forestry
www.fsc.org   FSC® C020056

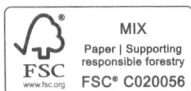

Image credits: Shutterstock: 12, 15, 122 / Epine;
4, 8, 18 / aniok; 6, 7, 16, 17, 27-29, 49, 51, 52, 54,
60, 61, 64, 66, 67, 69, 70, 72, 73, 76, 77, 88, 90, 97,
98, 105-107, 109, 120, 121, 124-126 / Foxyliam; 14,
94, 95, 98 / Tuleedin; 91, 93 / Avdeeva Ina; 10,
11, 16, 17, 26, 31-33, 35-37, 39, 41, 56-58, 74, 76,
77, 78, 80, 81-83, 84, 86, 87, 101, 103, 110, 111, 113,
115, 128 / Masha Dav; 116, 118 / HelenSun; 21, 23
cuttlefish84.

THE POCKET

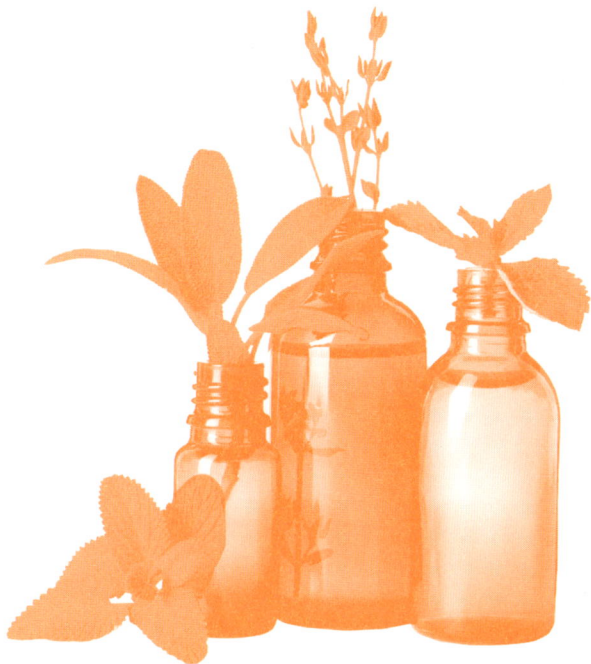

ESSENTIAL OILS

G:

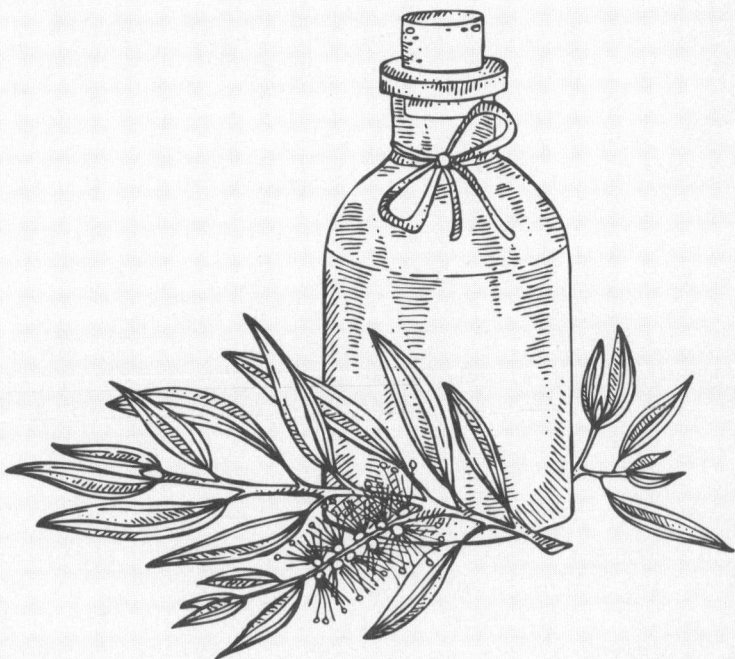

Introduction

Our sense of smell is linked powerfully to the mind and our emotions, and since the dawn of time, aromatic plants have been used by humankind in medicine, rituals, cooking and cosmetics. Essential oils are the concentrated fragrances of these plants in liquid form.

These oils have long been revered for their healing properties and have a wide range of therapeutic uses that support mind, body and spirit. They can ease certain symptoms, soothe or elevate mood and boost immunity, all while enveloping us in delicious and distinctive scents.

Read on to find out about 30 of the most popular essential oils today. Each one has its own profile, history, complementary oils and suggestions for use.

How to use essential oils

When you buy an essential oil, it is around a hundred times stronger than the oil found in the original plant. As such, it should always be treated with care and used in very small quantities, just a few drops at a time. Some popular ways to use these oils are:

Massage

One of the most effective methods of using essential oils is to add them to a carrier oil and use them in a massage. This way they are absorbed, in tiny amounts, through the skin for maximum therapeutic benefit. (*See page 8.*)

Bath oil

Add a few drops of a single oil, or blend of oils, to a tablespoon of a base oil and stir into your bath. Then lie back and inhale the vapours as you soak. You could also add a few drops of your favourite oil to a neutral body wash or shampoo.

Perfume burner or diffuser

Add a few drops of your favourite oil, or oils, to a diffuser or burner and enjoy being wrapped in the scent as it fills a room.

Room spray

To create a refreshing or relaxing atmosphere in a space, mix 30 drops of essential oil with 2 fl oz (60 ml) water in a small spray bottle, shake to combine and then spray liberally around the area.

Cotton balls

Add a few drops of oil to cotton balls and leave them around the home to gently suffuse the atmosphere with scent. This is especially popular with the oils that work as moth and insect repellents, such as patchouli, lemongrass and peppermint.

Massage with essential oils

Commonly called aromatherapy massage, this way of using essential oils combines their individual healing properties, usually in a blend of three oils, with the proven restorative benefits of respectful touch.

If making your own massage oil blends, always follow a "recipe" which indicates the correct number of drops of each oil to use – some are more powerful than others – and suggests a suitable carrier or base oil. Such oils include sweet almond, jojoba, avocado, argan and apricot kernel oil.

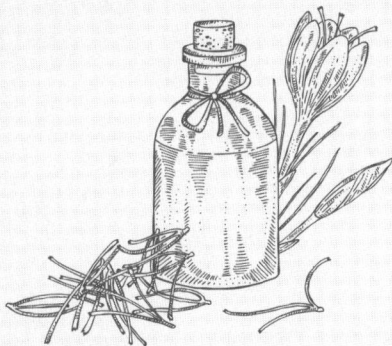

Sensitive skin massage

As with any massage, extra care should be taken with sensitive skin of any kind. When using essential oils for massage, use half the number of drops stated in the recipe in the same amount of carrier oil.

In addition, some oils, such as tea tree, ylang ylang, lemongrass and may chang, are deemed too strong for sensitive skin, so should be swapped with milder alternatives.

Always consult a healthcare professional before using essential oils for massage in pregnancy.

Extraction

Essential oils are extracted from their plants by three main processes.

STEAM DISTILLATION is the most common method. This is when large quantities of plant material are packed into a metal container called a still, before steam is pumped through it at high pressure.

This produces an aromatic steam which then passes through a cooling pipe and condenses back into water, with the oil floating on the top. This is then removed and bottled as the essential oil.

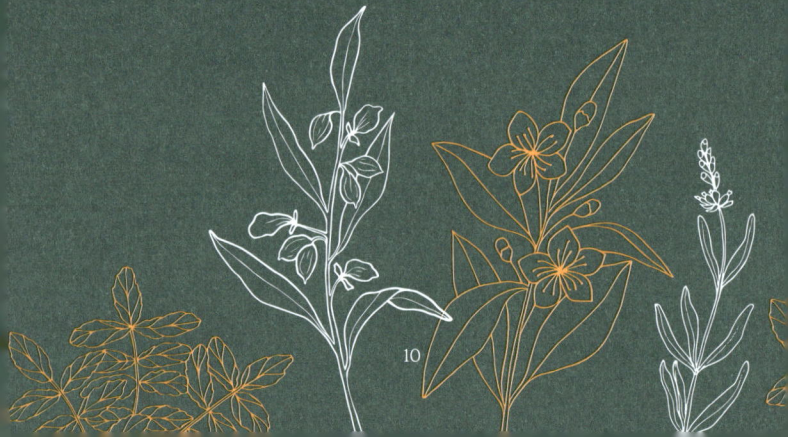

The other two methods of obtaining essential oil are expression and solvent extraction.

EXPRESSION is when oil is squeezed from the peel of citrus fruits, such as oranges, grapefruits and lemons.

SOLVENT EXTRACTION is the chemical process used to make oil from those flowers that are too delicate for steam distillation. The flowers are soaked in a solvent and then processed to give a thick and extremely concentrated oil. Such oils are called "absolutes" and are usually the most costly due to their complex and expensive extraction procedure.

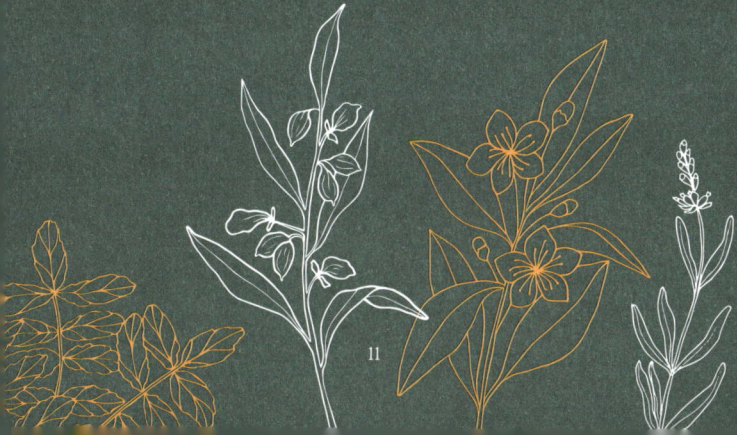

Quality essential oils

In the USA, essential oils are not regulated by the FDA. In the UK, some traders choose to be members of the Aromatherapy Trade Council, who conduct quality checks of their members.

In Australia, essential oils are regulated and are classified as industrial chemicals.

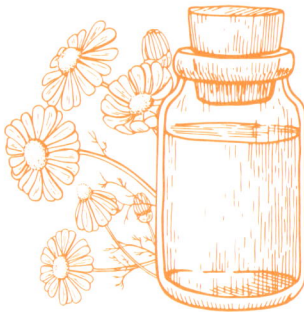

When purchasing essential oils, consider the below advice to ensure you are buying pure, quality oil:

🔸 Only buy 100 per cent pure essential oils – never with a mixing agent or added chemicals.

🔸 The extraction method and place of origin should be clearly labelled (if it is missing, question the provenance of the brand).

🔸 Check the botanical name of the oil is shown – this will tell you the exact source of the oil, as there may be more than one type of the plant.

🔸 Pure essential oils will be more expensive than synthetic oils, so ensure you are paying a sensible price for the quality you want. Remember, you will need to use less of a pure oil!

🔸 Buy oils in dark glass bottles: glass creates a natural oxygen barrier, and the dark colour protects from light and heat.

"Essential oils have a structure which only mother nature can put together. They have a life force, an additional impulse which can only be found in living things."

Robert Tisserand,
Aromatherapy (1988)

Storage

Always store your essential oils in dark glass bottles as this will protect the liquid from sunlight and UV damage. Pay attention to the storage instructions.

Most oils keep for around a year if stored in a cool, dark place, but will last for two years if kept in the refrigerator. Citrus oils are an exception to this and usually last for about half this time.

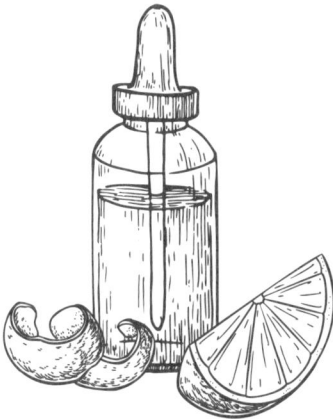

Alternative uses

As well as using essential oils in massage, bath oils or diffusers, try them around the home.

Cleaning

Certain essential oils are known for their antibacterial properties and can be added to a floor, surface or glass cleaner for an amazing scent and an extra boost. Add a few drops to your vacuum-cleaner bag or filter to spread a pleasant fragrance on your carpets and around the home, or in your waste bin to combat bad smells.

TRY: Eucalyptus, tea tree, lemongrass, lemon.

Laundry

Add a few drops of your favourite oil to your laundry load for freshly scented clothes. In addition, tea tree can be used in a cold soak with baking soda for heavily soiled items.

TRY: Lavender, tea tree, peppermint.

Bug and moth deterrent

Some oils are known for their bug-repellent properties, be that biting insects or fabric-hungry moths. A few drops of oil on cotton balls placed around the home or in drawers or wardrobes should do the trick.

TRY: Peppermint, patchouli, lemongrass, lavender.

A first-aid kit of oils

Such is the comfort and relief provided by essential oils that it's a great idea to have your own personal first-aid kit of your favourites to use when needed.

As well as the oils, a little bottle of carrier oil and a couple of small spray bottles will be useful. Staples for this kit might include the oils opposite.

Remember, essential oils are for external use only and should never be taken orally. If accidentally swallowed for any reason, seek medical help immediately.

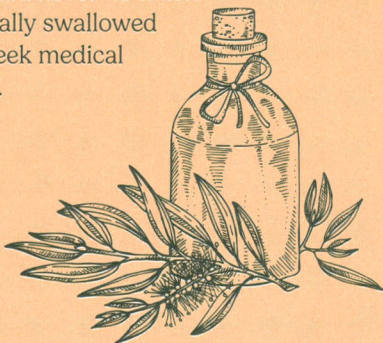

Lavender

For relaxation and to aid sleep. Add to a warm bath or make a room or pillow spray.

Peppermint

For headaches and nausea. A few drops on a cotton ball or tissue will clear and calm mind and body.

Patchouli or lemongrass

As an insect repellent. Used in an oil burner, on cotton balls or in a room spray to keep the bugs at bay.

Tea tree

As an antiseptic. Dilute with a small amount of carrier oil and apply to minor wounds.

"These remedies work, not by attacking disease, but by flooding our bodies with the beautiful vibrations of higher nature, in the presence of which dis-ease melts as snow in the sunshine."

Edward Bach,
Ye Suffer From Yourselves (1931)

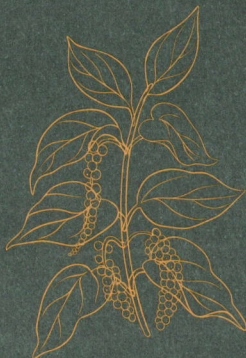

Black pepper

Piper Nigrum

MADE FROM:
Peppercorns

APPEARANCE:
Colourless

FRAGRANCE FAMILY:
Spicy

KEY AROMAS:
Warm, pungent, spicy

A kitchen staple as well as an oil, black pepper essential oil is made by steam distillation of the plant's unripe fruit – the peppercorns – which are dried in the sun and then crushed.

The world's most-traded spice, black pepper has been used for around 4,000 years, particularly in India and Southeast Asia where it grows in abundance. Such was its value that in ancient times it was known as "black gold".

Long-used in traditional Eastern medicine to treat digestive, circulatory and immune issues, black pepper essential oil is also used to comfort and calm a weary spirit and help combat insomnia.

This warm and powerful oil with woody undertones mixes well in a massage or bath oil blend with spicy, woody or citrus scents such as cardamom, rosemary, eucalyptus or lemongrass.

Black pepper uses

TONES CIRCULATORY SYSTEM
Eases aches, pains and stiffness; improves circulation.

SUPPORTS IMMUNITY
Builds defences against bacterial and viral infections.

BOOSTS DIGESTIVE SYSTEM
Aids a sluggish digestion and calms stomach cramps; revives appetite after illness.

SOOTHES MOOD
Comforts a tired or anxious spirit and lifts mood.

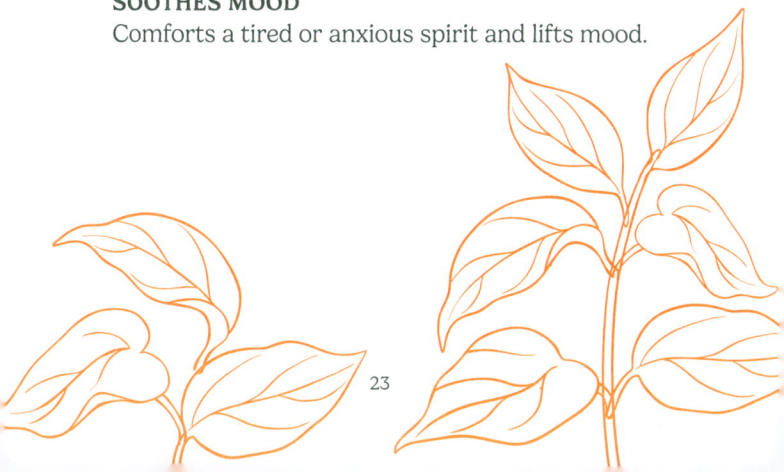

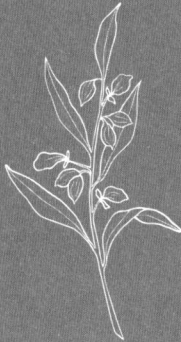

Cardamom

Elettaria cardamomum

MADE FROM:
Seeds

APPEARANCE:
Pale, almost colourless

FRAGRANCE FAMILY:
Spicy

KEY AROMAS:
Warm, rich, sweet, fruity

This aromatic spice belongs to the same family as ginger and has similar warming and uplifting properties.

Used in cooking and traditional medicine for at least 3,000 years, cardamom essential oil is made by steam distillation of the plant's small black seeds which are found in its distinctive hard seed pods.

Known for helping to treat immune, digestive and respiratory problems, it also soothes and cheers the mind, and its pods and seeds can be chewed to sweeten the breath.

Cardamom oil's distinctive fruity and spicy aroma with softer woody undertones mixes well with other spice oils, and with flower oils such as neroli and ylang ylang.

Cardamom uses

SETTLES DIGESTION
Regulates bowel habits; helps relieve constipation, stomach cramps and indigestion.

SOOTHES ANXIETY
Energizes lethargic feelings, settles anxiety and boosts mood.

BOOSTS IMMUNE SYSTEM
Nurtures and protects the body's natural defences.

AIDS RECUPERATION
Supports the body when recovering from illness, especially a viral or respiratory kind.

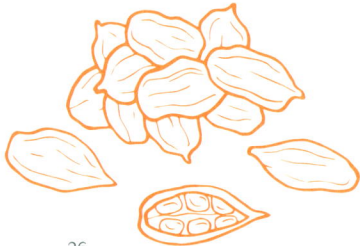

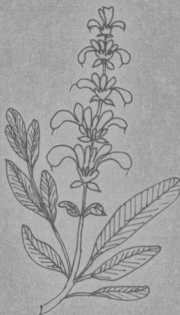

Clary sage

Salvia sclarea

MADE FROM:
Flowers and stalks

APPEARANCE:
Pale yellow

FRAGRANCE FAMILY:
Herbal

KEY AROMAS:
Rich, soft, musky, nutty

The largest of the sage family of plants, clary sage stands up to 4 ft (1.2 m) in height and has pretty pinkish-purple blooms from which the essential oil is extracted by steam distillation.

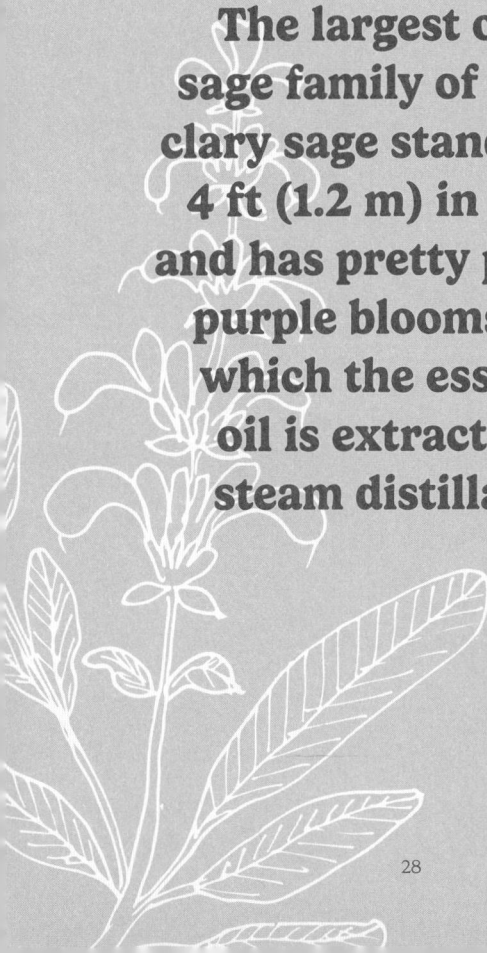

Clary sage has a powerful bouquet and is used widely in perfumery for its ability to give a scent a long-lasting aroma.

Its leaves have been used since at least the 17th century as a remedy for skin problems and the essential oil has similar skin-soothing properties in a massage oil or bath blend.

Chiefly used today to support regulation of the menstrual cycle and associated hormones, clary sage also has a gentle sedative effect and can restore balance in an emotional or stressful time.

Clary sage's strong, musky notes mix well with woody scents, such as sandalwood, frankincense and cypress, and with rose and citrus aromas.

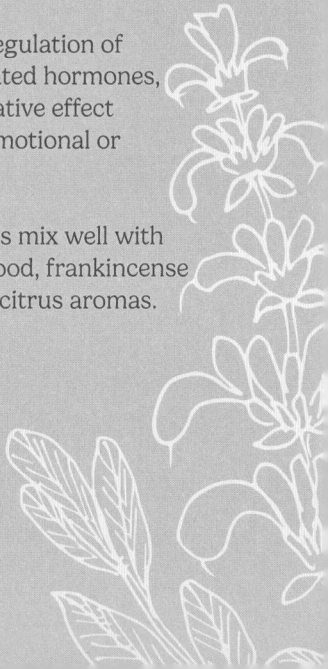

Clary sage uses

BALANCES HORMONES
Helps regulate the menstrual cycle and relieve painful period cramps.

REGULATES SKIN
Balances out hormonal skin, especially greasy or oily skin.

LIFTS MOOD
Eases anxiety, feelings of overwhelm or irritability and mood swings.

SOOTHES MUSCLES
Reduces cramps and spasms in digestive or respiratory systems.

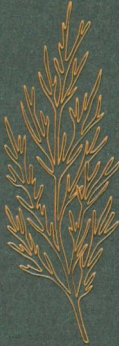

Cypress

Cupressus sempervirens

MADE FROM:
Leaves and young branches

APPEARANCE:
Yellow

FRAGRANCE FAMILY:
Woody

KEY AROMAS:
Warm, woody, sweet

Cypress trees have been around for millions of years and some specimens alive today are known to be more than 2,000 years old.

The ancient Greeks used their leaves to treat wounds, and burned cypress branches to purify the air during cremations.

Cypress essential oil comes from an evergreen tree native to the Eastern Mediterranean and is extracted from its twigs and leaves via steam distillation.

The cypress has been a symbol of mourning since Greek and Roman times. In mythology, handsome young Cyparissus, a favourite of Apollo, accidentally killed a beautiful stag. Distraught, he asked Apollo to enable him to weep forever. Apollo turned him into a cypress tree and the tree's sap represents the tears of Cyparissus.

This strongly aromatic oil with smoky and spicy undertones mixes well with a combination of other deep oils, such as cardamom or clary sage, and citrus scents such as grapefruit or orange.

Cypress uses

SUPPORTS MENSTRUAL HEALTH
Regulates the cycle and supports female hormones.

SOOTHES THE MIND
Calms tension and reduces overwhelm.

RESTORES THE SPIRITS
Often used in meditation and for periods of transition and new beginnings.

BOOSTS SKIN, CIRCULATION AND RESPIRATION
Tones the skin, revitalizes the circulation and soothes sore coughs.

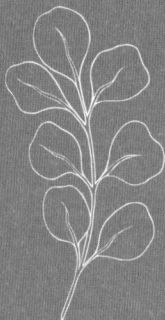

Eucalyptus

Eucalyptus globulus

MADE FROM:
Leaves and young twigs

APPEARANCE:
Colourless

FRAGRANCE FAMILY:
Woody

KEY AROMAS:
Sharp, medicinal, green, deep,
woody, clearing

The refreshing aroma of eucalyptus is said to clear the mind, aid concentration, boost energy and dissolve negative feelings. Its oil is extracted from the leaves and twigs via steam distillation.

A long-standing traditional remedy in Australia and New Zealand, an infusion of eucalyptus leaves gives off a cleansing vapour that eases congestion and is also used as an antiseptic wash for bites, cuts and grazes.

Eucalyptus blends well with other evergreen oils, such as tea tree or cedarwood, combined with sweeter or citrus notes, such as may chang, lemon or mandarin.

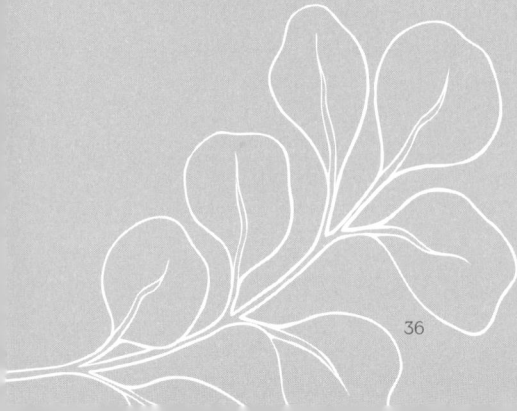

Native to Australia, the evergreen eucalyptus with its green-grey leaves has a pleasant, invigorating scent with strong hints of camphor.

Eucalyptus uses

CLEARS CONGESTION
Acts as a nasal and chest decongestant; helps
ward off colds and flu.

STIMULATES THE MIND
Aids concentration, clarifies and refreshes,
dissipates negative emotions.

RELIEVES SORE MUSCLES
Eases muscle pulls and sprains; stimulates
blood flow to warm cold hands and feet.

ACTS AS AN ANTIBACTERIAL CLEANER
Add to hot water for cleaning floors and
surfaces around the home.

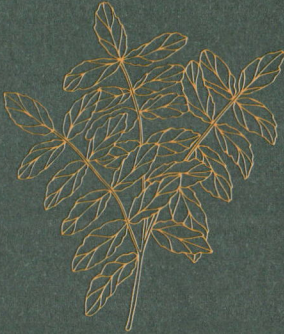

Frankincense

Boswellia carterii

MADE FROM:
Tree resin

APPEARANCE:
Pale yellow

FRAGRANCE FAMILY:
Balsamic

KEY AROMAS:
Warm, sharp, resinous, fresh

Frankincense trees grow in inhospitable desert or mountain regions of the Middle East and Africa. Their bark is scored to release milky resin that hardens into small pieces known as tears. This resin is ground and steam-distilled to produce the essential oil.

Its aroma – and perhaps its association with the Divine and places of worship – inspires a state of deep reflection, but its oil is also incredibly nourishing for the skin.

Frankincense's distinctive notes, which begin with sharp, resinous tones before becoming richer and sweeter as it evaporates, blend well with other rich scents such as rose, neroli, sandalwood and ginger.

Frankincense has
been used as a medicinal
oil and as incense since
ancient times, and was
one of the gifts brought
by the Magi to the infant
Christ, symbolizing
his divinity. It is
widely burned in many
traditional churches
to this day.

Frankincense uses

NOURISHES SKIN
Restores tired or sun-damaged skin, rejuvenates mature skin and improves the appearance of fine lines.

CALMS EMOTIONS
Provides an excellent aid for meditation; uplifts the mood.

SUPPORTS HEALTHY RESPIRATION
Soothes coughs; encourages calming and deepening of the breath.

BOOSTS IMMUNITY
Supports resistance to infections.

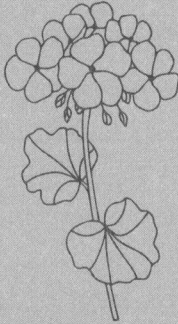

Geranium

Pelargonium graveolens

MADE FROM:
Leaves

APPEARANCE:
Pale yellow

FRAGRANCE FAMILY:
Floral

KEY AROMAS:
Intensely floral, green, fresh,
sweet and rosy

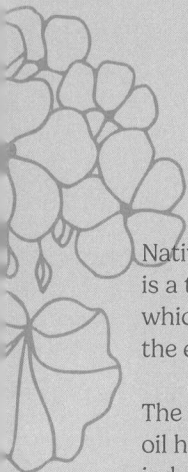

Native to southern Africa, this geranium species is a tropical plant with rose-scented leaves, which are picked when young and turned into the essential oil by steam distillation.

The intense rosy scent of geranium essential oil has made it a staple in the perfume industry for many years and it is one of the most common ingredients used in perfume and perfumed products.

Soothing and uplifting, geranium oil promotes a state of relaxation and works wonders on all types of skin.

This soft, sweet and rosy oil has a lightness that makes it popular for facials. It blends well with a combination of deeper scents, such as frankincense and sandalwood, and sharper citrus notes, such as may chang and neroli.

Geranium uses

BALANCES HORMONES
Soothes menstrual symptoms, particularly PMS and fluid retention.

REGULATES EMOTIONS
Combats negativity; eases emotional stress.

PROMOTES HEALTHY SKIN
Heals and repairs dry skin; balances skin that is too oily or too dry.

SOOTHES DIGESTION
Eases stomach cramps and general discomfort.

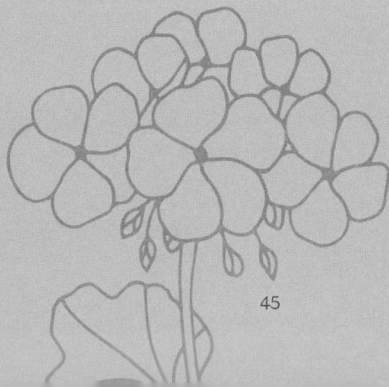

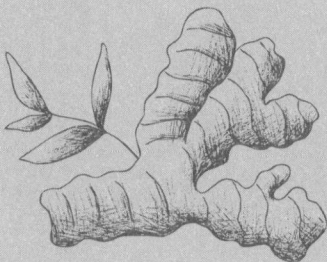

Ginger

Zingiber officinale

MADE FROM:
Dried roots

APPEARANCE:
Almost colourless

FRAGRANCE FAMILY:
Spicy

KEY AROMAS:
Warm, sharp, rich, spicy, deep

Native to Southeast Asia, ginger is a tropical flowering plant with nobbly bulbous roots that are dried and steam-distilled to produce an essential oil that is much sweeter smelling than fresh ginger root.

Used in cookery and medicine for thousands of years, ginger has become a staple ingredient in kitchens everywhere and is used worldwide as a remedy for colds, flu and indigestion.

Its spicy, clean but warm flavours and aroma boosts energy, especially during illness, while soothing and calming body and mind.

A powerful oil, ginger should be used sparingly in blends, but works well with a mix of woody, spicy, smoky and citrusy scents, such as cardamom, cedarwood, lemon and sweet orange.

Ginger uses

SOOTHES DIGESTION
Eases cramps, constipation and indigestion.

BOOSTS IMMUNITY
Builds protection against viral and
bacterial illness.

SUPPORTS THE EMOTIONS
Helps release tension; acts as a soothing
emotional balm.

STIMULATES THE CIRCULATION
Relieves tired muscles, warms limbs and
cold hands and feet.

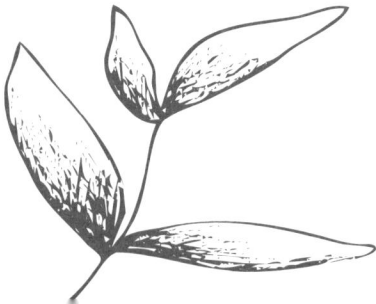

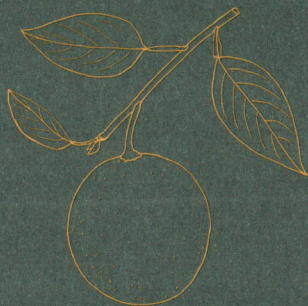

Grapefruit

Citrus x paradisi

MADE FROM:
Fruit peel

APPEARANCE:
Pale orange

FRAGRANCE FAMILY:
Citrus

KEY AROMAS:
Sharp, zesty, refreshing, bright

The evergreen grapefruit tree with its shiny leaves and white, star-shaped flowers thrives in sunny climes and can grow up to 30 ft (10 m) in height. Its large round fruit have thick yellow peel from which its essential oil is expressed.

Stimulating and uplifting, the scent of grapefruit is bitter-sweet and its flavouring is widely used in food and drink products and cosmetics. It is cleansing and detoxifying, both on the palette and in its oil form, and brightens and cheers body and mind.

This zesty, fresh oil with an underlying sweet note blends well with scents that have a similar sharpness but also have an earthiness for balance. Try it with fennel, cardamom, tea tree, ginger or juniper berry.

Grapefruit uses

PROMOTES MENTAL STIMULATION
Improves concentration and boosts mood.

CLEANSES SKIN
Tones and cleanses; its astringent qualities
are particularly good for oily skin.

DETOXIFIES THE SYSTEM
Acts as a natural diuretic and helps to remove
impurities from the body.

LIFTS MOOD
Improves confidence and encourages positivity;
eases symptoms of PMS.

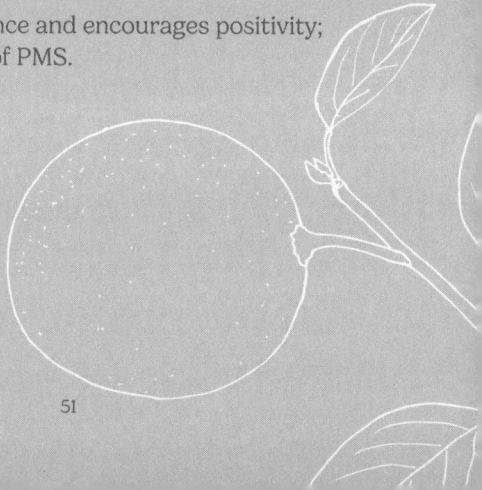

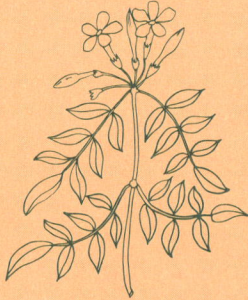

Jasmine absolute

Jasminum officinale

MADE FROM:
Flowers

APPEARANCE:
Medium consistency and golden
orange-yellow to brown in colour

FRAGRANCE FAMILY:
Floral

KEY AROMAS:
Sweet, floral, heady, musky, soft

Jasmine is a pretty, deciduous climbing plant with deep green leaves and star-shaped white flowers that exude an intense, intoxicating fragrance.

Jasmine flowers are too delicate for steam distillation so their oil is extracted by diluting them in a solvent which produces a highly concentrated, or "absolute", oil.

This highly nourishing oil is wonderful for the skin and promotes a deep sense of wellbeing and sensuality; as such, it is also well known for its aphrodisiacal properties.

The potent floral, musky scent of jasmine blends well with other powerful aromas such as rose, frankincense and neroli, or sweet orange and sandalwood.

Jasmine flowers bloom and release their perfume at dusk, so are picked at night with each one producing a tiny amount of oil.

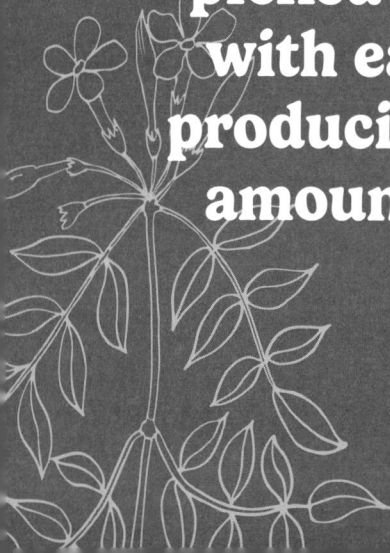

Jasmine uses

BOOSTS MOOD
Eases anxiety and improves confidence.

HEALS SKIN
Rejuvenates dry or ageing skin; improves elasticity and reduces the appearance of wrinkles.

ACTS AS AN APHRODISIAC
Supports a healthy libido and encourages intimacy.

SUPPORTS MENSTRUAL HEALTH
Regulates cycle and relieves period pain.

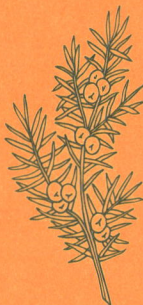

Juniper berry

Juniperus communis

MADE FROM:
Berries

APPEARANCE:
Thin, colourless

FRAGRANCE FAMILY:
Green

KEY AROMAS:
Fresh, green, woody, peppery;
sweeter and softer as it evaporates

Long valued for its purifying properties, juniper was burned as incense in ancient Greece and used in ancient Egypt as part of the mummification process.

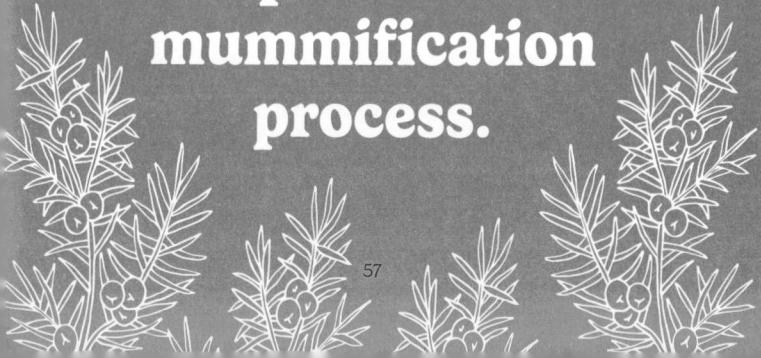

Juniper is a prickly evergreen shrub with small green berries that ripen to a purple-black colour over 18 months. Its essential oil is extracted from the dark berries by steam distillation.

Juniper berries are famously used to flavour gin as well as being a popular ingredient in jams, sauces and stuffings, particularly in Central and Eastern Europe.

A powerful oil, juniper should be used with care, often in tiny amounts, but blends well with woody scents, such as cypress and rosemary, as well as oils with citrus notes, such as myrtle, lemon and petitgrain.

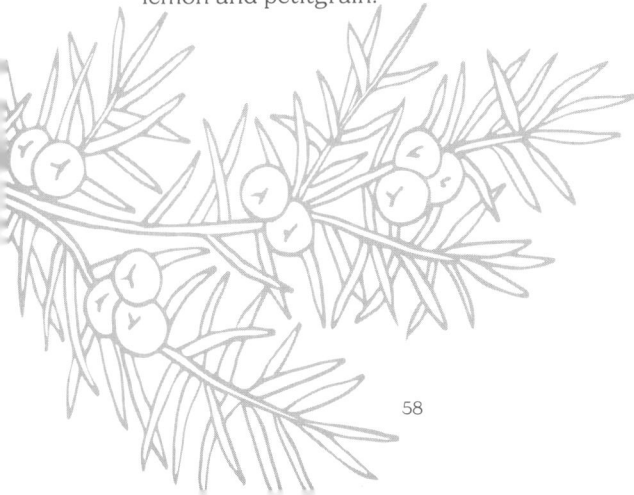

Juniper berry uses

SHARPENS THE MIND
Eases mental tiredness and improves focus.

DETOXIFIES
Helps remove excess fluid from the system with its diuretic properties.

SUPPORTS THE CIRCULATION
Boosts blood flow; warms cold hands and feet; soothes muscle aches; relieves symptoms of arthritis.

LIFTS THE SPIRITS
Purges negative feelings and lightens emotional baggage.

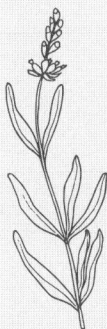

Lavender

Lavandula angustifolia

MADE FROM:
Stalks and flowering tops

APPEARANCE:
Pale, almost colourless

FRAGRANCE FAMILY:
Woody aromatic

KEY AROMAS:
Floral, fresh, sweet, warm, pungent

Many lavender varieties are grown around the world and the oil's aroma can be floral or sharper and more medicinal depending on its source.

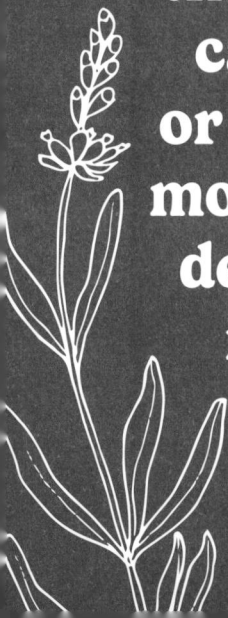

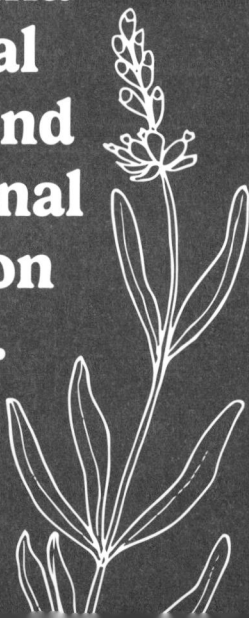

Perhaps the most commonly used essential oil, lavender is made from steam distillation of the purple flowers and stalks of this popular bushy shrub.

Lavender has long been known for its healing properties, which range from antiseptic, anti-inflammatory and pain-relieving to deeply calming, relaxing and soporific.

This oil's highly aromatic, mildly medicinal scent blends well with warm floral and citrus fragrances, such as lemon, neroli and rosewood, along with herbal and spicy oils, such as tea tree and cardamom.

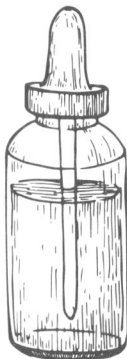

Lavender uses

HEALS SKIN
Heals cuts, grazes, insect bites and minor burns
with its antiseptic properties; soothes sun-
damaged skin and promotes skin cell renewal.

AIDS RELAXATION
Calms mood; helps promote restful and
rejuvenating sleep.

RELIEVES PAIN
Alleviates muscular aches and pains, headaches
and menstrual pain.

SUPPORTS HEALTHY RESPIRATION
Soothes these body systems and fights cold
and flu symptoms.

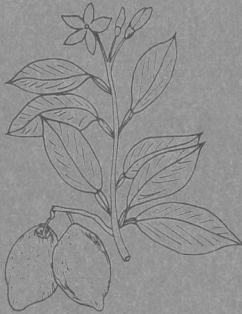

Lemon

Citrus limonum

MADE FROM:
Fruit peel

APPEARANCE:
Thin, yellow

FRAGRANCE FAMILY:
Citrus

KEY AROMAS:
Sharp, fruity, zesty, bright

Squeezed from the fruit peel of the evergreen citrus tree, lemon oil is mostly produced in Italy, Florida and California where these plants thrive. A healthy tree can produce more than a thousand lemons in a single year.

Lemons are used worldwide in cooking – the juice flavours drinks and sweets, is used in sauces and tenderizes meats, while preserved whole lemons appear in many savoury Mediterranean and North African dishes.

The clean, purifying properties of lemon oil are gently invigorating for body, mind and spirit, brightening mood and giving rise to feelings of contentment.

A zesty, bright oil, with hints of sweetness and sherbet as it evaporates, lemon blends well with woody and fruity oils, such as cypress, rosemary, juniper and geranium, and also works well with peppermint to blow away the cobwebs!

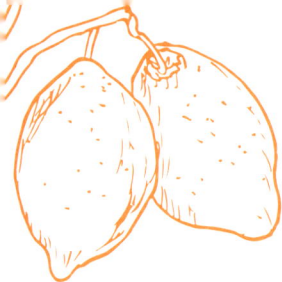

Lemon uses

LIFTS MOOD
Alleviates low spirits, boosts confidence and soothes anxiety.

CLEANSES SKIN
Tones and balances skin, especially if excessively oily.

TONES THE CIRCULATION
Invigorates tired muscles and improves energy.

DETOXIFIES
Stimulates the lymphatic system to help purify the body of toxins; boosts immunity.

FREASHENS THE AIR
Cleanses air of impurities and bad smells.

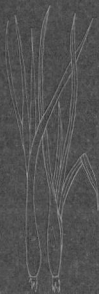

Lemongrass

Cymbopogon citratus

MADE FROM:
Grass leaves and stems

APPEARANCE:
Thin, pale yellow

FRAGRANCE FAMILY:
Citrus

KEY AROMAS:
Sweet yet sharp, zesty, sherbet-like,
powerful, lemony

A fragrant tropical grass with sharp, blade-like leaves up to 5 ft (1.5 m) tall, lemongrass yields its pale oil by steam distillation.

Widely used in cooking and as a traditional remedy in its native South and Southeast Asia, lemongrass adds a fragrant, spicy taste to many dishes and treats headaches, fevers, muscle aches and inflammation.

Invigorating and uplifting, it restores energy and boosts the circulation, and its fresh lemony perfume creates a peaceful, clear atmosphere around the home.

Lemongrass is a powerful oil with a strong citrus and grassy aroma. It blends well with floral woody oils, such as patchouli, myrtle and lavender, and with spicy scents, such as turmeric and cardamom.

Lemongrass uses

STABILIZES MOOD
Calms fraught nerves; revives mental tiredness.

SUPPORTS GOOD DIGESTION
Stimulates a sluggish system and
relieves constipation.

SOOTHES MUSCLES
Reduces stiffness, aches and pains by boosting
circulation in affected areas.

REPELS INSECTS
Wards off mosquitos and other biting insects.

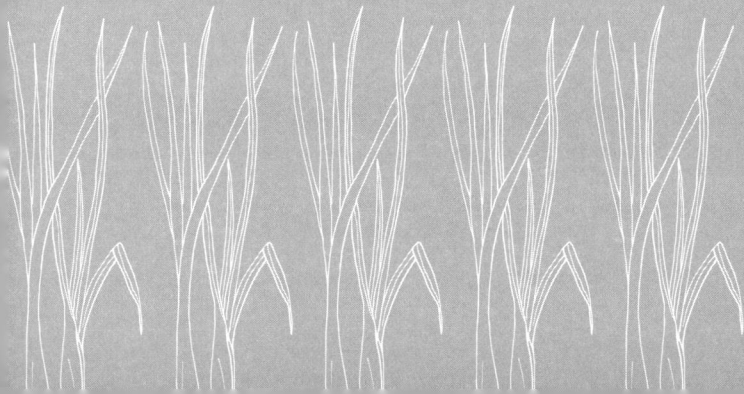

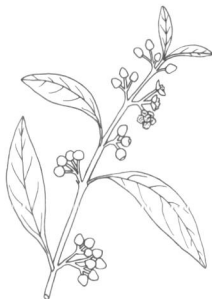

May chang

Litsea cubeba

MADE FROM:
Small peppercorn-like fruits

APPEARANCE:
Thin and pale yellow

FRAGRANCE FAMILY:
Fruity

KEY AROMAS:
Light, sweet, lemon sherbet, citrusy
with spicy undertones

Native to China, this small aromatic tree from the tropics has lemon-scented, fine, soft leaves and small, peppercorn-like fruits. Sometimes called the "mountain pepper", its oil is extracted from the fruit by steam distillation.

May chang is used widely in the perfume business in soaps and scents, and also as a spicy, lemony flavour in foods.

A feature of traditional remedies for treating headaches, fevers, aches and respiratory issues, may chang also has a gently uplifting and cheering effect and is good for calming anxiety.

Despite its lemon sherbet aroma, may chang is milder than lemongrass and sweeter and softer than lemon oil. It blends well with floral scents such as rose, lavender and sweet orange, alongside woody fragrances, such as cedarwood, myrtle and frankincense.

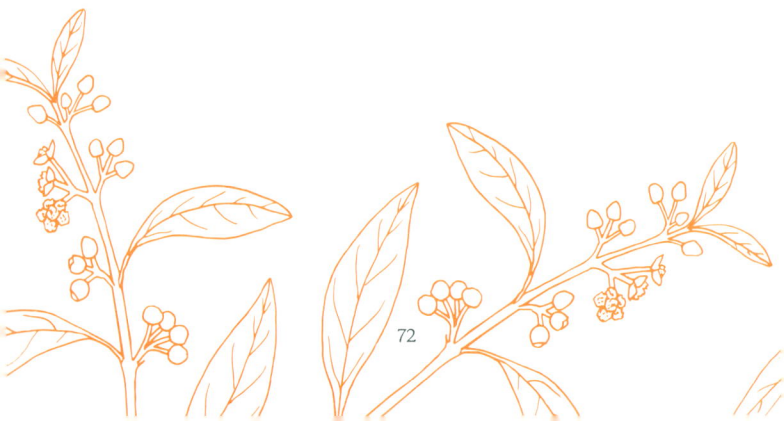

May Chang uses

REVIVES MUSCLES
Relieves stiffness, tired muscles and general aches and pains.

LIFTS EMOTIONS
Refreshes mental energy, restores vitality and clears the mind.

BOOSTS IMMUNITY
Supports the heart, digestive and circulatory systems.

TONES SKIN
Balances and tones oily and combination skin.

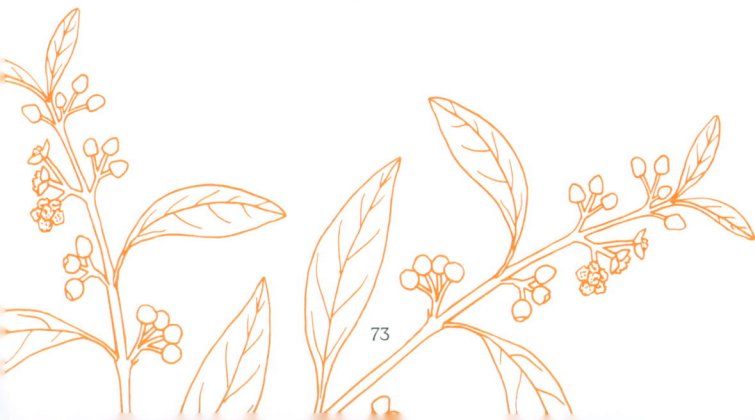

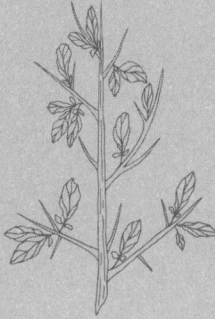

Myrrh

Commiphora myrrha

MADE FROM:
Plant gum

APPEARANCE:
Pale yellow

FRAGRANCE FAMILY:
Balsamic

KEY AROMAS:
Sharp, medicinal (sometimes called "bitter"),
smoky, warm, becoming sweeter

Myrrh is a thorny desert bush with small green leaves and white flowers. Its oil is extracted by steam distillation of myrrh gum-resin, which is harvested by cutting incisions in the stem of the plant to release the sticky yellow gum.

Its name means "bitter" in Arabic, and there is a sharpness to its odour which can be described this way.

Myrrh's medicinal properties help treat a wide range of physical and emotional complaints. It has antibacterial and antiseptic qualities, reduces inflammation, relaxes the mind, restores the skin and generally brings feelings of warmth and comfort.

The highly aromatic myrrh has an unusual fragrance and blends well with a mix of woody and floral scents, such as vetiver, sandalwood, frankincense, neroli and rose.

One of the gifts brought by the Magi to the infant Christ, myrrh has been prized since antiquity as a sacred oil used to anoint kings, which is why the Magi deemed it a suitable offering.

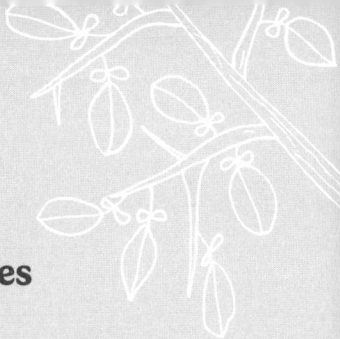

Myrrh uses

REPAIRS SKIN
Helps restore damaged skin, reduce
inflammation and heal wounds.

COMFORTS THE MIND
Calms an agitated mind and soothes anxiety
and tension.

SUPPORTS MENSTRUAL HEALTH
Eases cramps and gently balances mood swings.

SOOTHES CHEST
Settles coughs and warms and calms the
bronchial system.

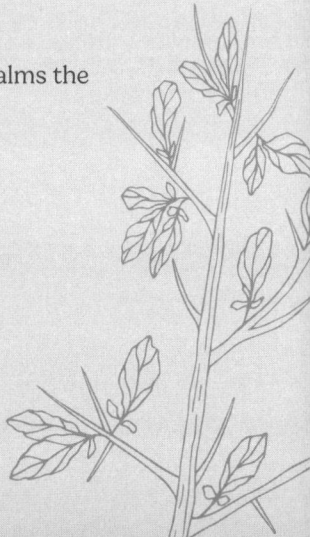

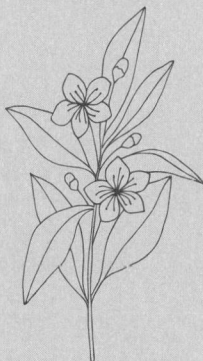

Myrtle

Myrtus communis

MADE FROM:
Leaves and twigs

APPEARANCE:
Pale yellow or greenish

FRAGRANCE FAMILY:
Woody

KEY AROMAS:
Fresh, green, sharp and citrusy

An aromatic shrub from the southern Mediterranean, myrtle has a reddish bark and small, green lance-shaped leaves from which the essential oil is extracted by steam distillation.

In ancient Greece, myrtle was burned as incense on altars dedicated to Aphrodite, goddess of love. Fragrant sprigs of myrtle are still often incorporated into wedding bouquets because of this association.

Myrtle has been drunk as a herbal tea remedy in the Mediterranean for centuries to support a healthy menstrual cycle, and steam from bowls of myrtle leaves boiled in water has been inhaled to ease congestion.

The gentle woody notes of myrtle combined with a fresh citrus aroma that sweetens on evaporation makes this oil blend well with other woody and floral scents, such as frankincense, myrrh, cedarwood, rose, geranium and neroli.

Myrtle uses

BOOSTS IMMUNE SYSTEM
Improves resistance to winter colds.

LIFTS MOOD
Calms anxiety and tension caused by stress.

TONES SKIN
Balances the skin and its astringent qualities can stabilize oily complexions. Also good for mature skin.

SOOTHES RESPIRATORY SYSTEM
Eases irritation from coughs.

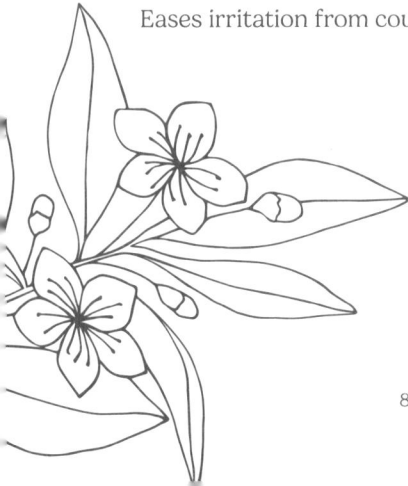

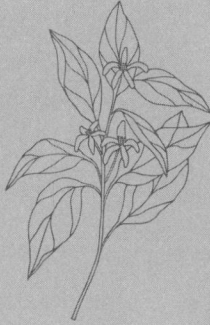

Neroli

Citrus x aurantium var. amara

MADE FROM:
Flowers

APPEARANCE:
Thin and pale yellow

FRAGRANCE FAMILY:
Floral

KEY AROMAS:
Rich, sweet, citrus, floral, woody,
spicy, orange

Neroli essential oil is made by steam distillation of the creamy white flowers of the bitter orange tree, which are picked at sunrise to best preserve their aroma.

The oil got its name when Anne Marie Orsini, Princess of Nerola, Italy, made it fashionable in the late 17th century as she used bitter orange essence to perfume her gloves and her bath.

One of the most popular and widely used essential oils, neroli lasts a long time on the skin and bestows a great sense of wellbeing. This can be uplifting, when its mix of bitter-sweet and floral notes are combined with citrus scents, such as lemon or sweet orange, or relaxing when blended with woody and resinous oils, such as sandalwood, frankincense and myrrh.

Neroli uses

BOOSTS MOOD
Works against feelings of despondency and
lifts the spirits.

BALANCES THE EMOTIONS
Eases feelings of anxiety and stress;
quietens panic.

CALMS THE DIGESTION
Soothes indigestion, feelings of nausea
and IBS symptoms.

RESTORES SKIN
Supports dry skin and revitalizes
the complexion.

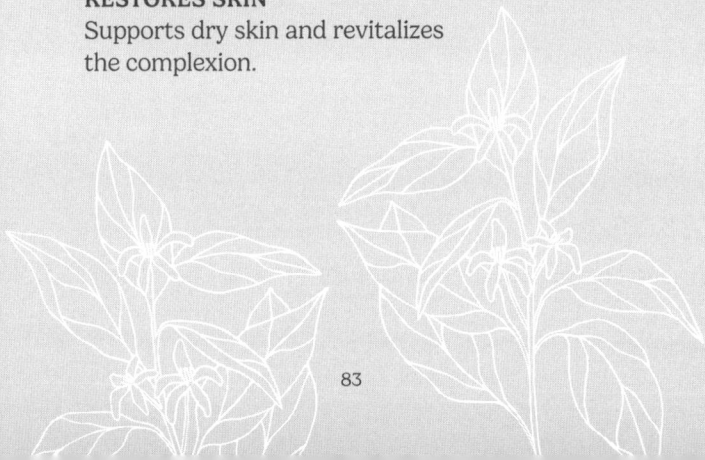

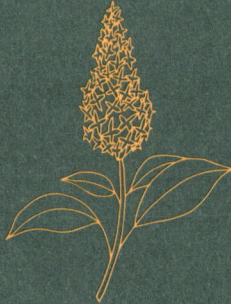

Patchouli

Pogostemon cablin

MADE FROM:
Leaves

APPEARANCE:
Thick with an amber colour

FRAGRANCE FAMILY:
Woody

KEY AROMAS:
Woody, musky and floral, with earthy
and smoky tones

A bushy perennial herb native to Southeast Asia, the patchouli plant is cultivated for its oil, which is extracted from the partially dried leaves by steam distillation.

Considered by many to be an aphrodisiac, patchouli's distinctive strong scent became hugely popular in the counter-cultural movement of the 1960s and '70s, and remains familiar to many as a result.

Patchouli oil's sensual musky aroma with its smoky undertones blends well with a mix of floral and resinous scents, such as jasmine, rose, lavender, frankincense and myrrh.

A traditional remedy in the East since ancient times, dried patchouli leaves are used to treat headaches, colds and nausea, and to protect precious material from moths.

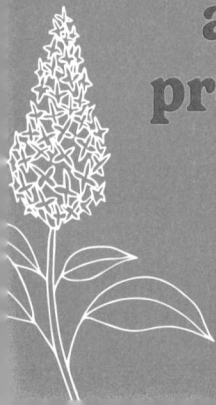

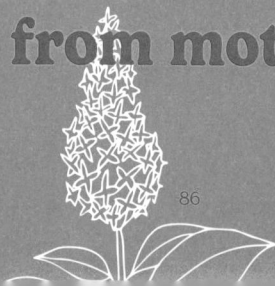

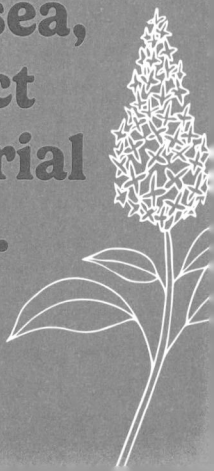

Patchouli uses

CALMS THE EMOTIONS
Grounds the spirit; combats stress and lack of confidence.

ACTS AS AN APHRODISIAC
Connects body and mind with a powerful sensual awareness.

TONES AND HEALS SKIN
Moisturizes dry or dull skin; heals damaged areas.

REPELS INSECTS
Wards off insects and protects clothes from moths.

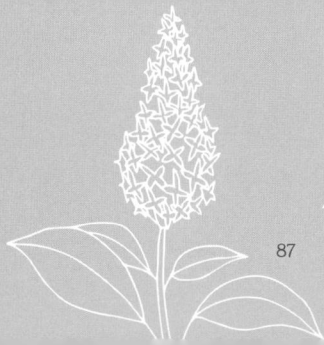

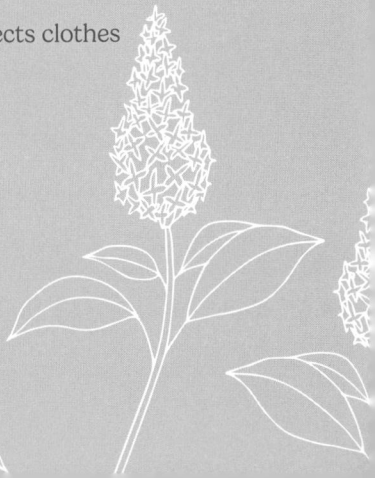

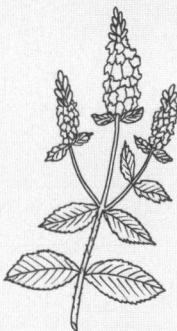

Peppermint

Mentha x piperita

MADE FROM:
Leaves

APPEARANCE:
Thin, very pale

FRAGRANCE FAMILY:
Minty

KEY AROMAS:
Minty, fresh, spicy, menthol, sweet

Widely drunk as a tea and used to flavour confectionery and toothpaste, peppermint is a vigorous herb with spiky clumps of pale purple flowers and dark green leaves which produce its essential oil via steam distillation.

Best known as a natural remedy to ease digestion and relieve headache pain, peppermint also lifts the spirits and restores lost energy.

An effective natural alternative to chemical insect repellents, peppermint has long been used to deter spiders and other bugs. Add a couple of drops to cotton-wool balls and place them around the home to ward off such unwanted visitors.

A powerful oil, peppermint is best avoided on the face, but it works well with ginger for digestive conditions and with may chang and rosemary to soothe the head, revive the mind and clear away brain fog.

Peppermint uses

RELIEVES HEADACHES
Cools and soothes headaches and migraine.

REFRESHES BODY AND MIND
Stimulates the senses; improves concentration
and memory.

TONES THE DIGESTIVE SYSTEM
Soothes indigestion; relieves nausea
and travel sickness.

CLEANSES THE RESPIRATORY SYSTEM
Clears blocked sinuses;
aids sinusitis.

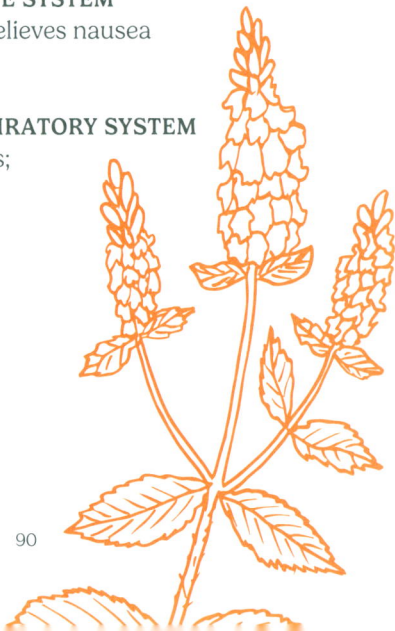

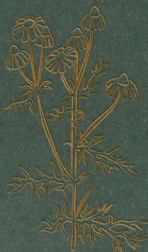

Roman chamomile

Anthemis nobilis

MADE FROM:
Flowers and stalks

APPEARANCE:
Thin and very pale greenish-blue

FRAGRANCE FAMILY:
Fruity

KEY AROMAS:
Sweet, fruity, herbaceous,
fresh, apple-like

Roman chamomile has soft green feathery leaves and small daisy-like flowers, which are picked, along with their stalks, and made into essential oil by steam distillation.

One of the oldest recorded medicinal herbs, it was used as a cure for fever in ancient Egypt, and has been a staple traditional remedy for a range of ailments for thousands of years. Particularly known for its calming effects, both on the mind and the digestion, it's no surprise that Roman chamomile is also beneficial for insomnia.

This sweet, herby oil with hints of apple blends well with other sweet scents, such as lavender and neroli, combined with spicier, earthier fragrances, such as ginger or sandalwood.

Chamomile uses

CALMS NERVES
Reduces stress and anxiety, soothes irritability
and helps combat insomnia.

EASES INFLAMMATION
Calms dry, inflamed or damaged skin.

SOOTHES STOMACH
Aids smooth digestion, eases nausea
and indigestion.

RELIEVES PAIN
Reduces muscle aches and stomach cramps,
relieves headaches.

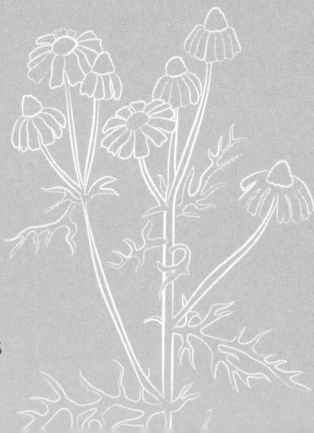

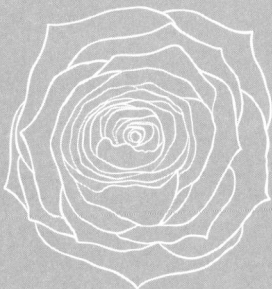

Rose absolute

Rosa centifolia

MADE FROM:
Flowers

APPEARANCE:
Thin and yellow-orange

FRAGRANCE FAMILY:
Floral

KEY AROMAS:
Floral, musky, rich

One of the two types of rose essential oil, rose absolute is produced from the large scented flowers of the *centifolia* or cabbage rose plant by solvent extraction.

Used in perfumery and cosmetics for thousands of years, rose absolute has an exquisite fragrance. This makes it perennially popular in skin treatments that combine its luxurious scent and healing properties to rejuvenate damaged skin, including broken capillaries and mild scarring.

This oil's soft but strong rosy aroma, with hints of musky sweetness, blends especially well with a combination of citrus and woody scents, such as lemon and vetiver, to soothe fraught emotions and bring peace.

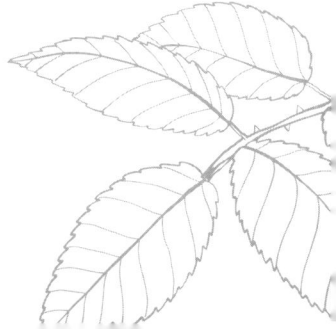

Rose absolute uses

HYDRATES SKIN
Softens and supports, especially dry or mature skin; boosts the complexion and combats sun damage.

BALANCES HORMONES
Supports menstrual symptoms such as fluid retention and PMS.

EASES INFLAMMATION
Soothes irritated skin and relieves muscle pain.

CALMS OVERWHELM
Helps with grief and heartache.

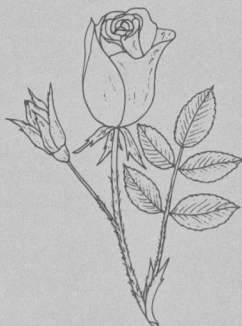

Rose otto

Rosa damascena

MADE FROM:
Flowers

APPEARANCE:
Thin and colourless

FRAGRANCE FAMILY:
Floral

KEY AROMAS:
Soft, rich and floral

It takes more
than 200 flowers to
produce a single
drop of rose otto
essential oil via steam
distillation, making it
one of the finest and
most expensive
oils there is.

Softer in scent than rose absolute, rose otto oil is made from the flowers of the damask rose in a labour-intensive process that involves harvesting the petals at sunrise when their fragrance is most powerful.

A popular ingredient in cooking, as well as cosmetics and perfume, rose water and petals from the damask rose are found in many Middle Eastern and Indian dishes, adding a depth and delicate floral note to spicy dishes.

Rose otto oil's exquisite rosy scent, with hints of citrus and honey, blends well with equally deep scents, such as sandalwood and frankincense, for a skin treat and an emotional lift. Alternatively, try mixing with herbal and citrusy scents, such as sweet orange and clary sage, for a calming blend to balance out any hormonal swings.

Rose otto uses

SOOTHES INFLAMMATION
Calms inflamed or irritated skin, aids repair
of minor burns.

BOOSTS MOOD
Nurtures, comforts and lifts the mood.

HYDRATES SKIN
Softens and supports, especially dry or mature
skin, boosting complexion and combatting
sun damage.

BALANCES HORMONES
Use during menstrual cycle to ease
unpleasant symptoms.

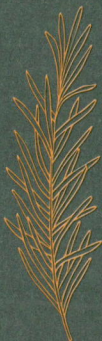

Rosemary

Rosmarinus officinalis

MADE FROM:
Leaves

APPEARANCE:
Colourless

FRAGRANCE FAMILY:
Woody

KEY AROMAS:
Fresh, enlivening, green, herbal,
with woody undertones

A popular aromatic herb in cooking, rosemary is a woody Mediterranean shrub packed with essential oil, which is extracted from its leaves by steam distillation.

It has been used since ancient times in medicinal remedies for aches, pains and rheumatism, and was burned as an incense, especially in sick rooms, to purify the air with its powerful herbal and camphorous scent.

In the language of plants, rosemary is another that has traditionally featured in wedding bouquets since the Middle Ages, said to symbolize fidelity between the bride and groom.

Stimulating and uplifting for the mind, the revitalizing scent of rosemary oil blends well with similarly fresh scents such as lemon, eucalyptus, black pepper and peppermint.

Rosemary is commonly harvested in midsummer when its oil is most highly concentrated.

Rosemary uses

IMPROVES CIRCULATION
Warms the skin and stimulates circulation, especially on the scalp, making it a good hair tonic.

STIMULATES THE MIND
Energizes and refreshes the mind; clears mental tiredness and boosts enthusiasm.

EASES CONGESTION
Relieves respiratory distress caused by colds, flu and allergies; provides a natural expectorant.

RELIEVES PAIN
Anti-inflammatory; eases joint and muscle pain.

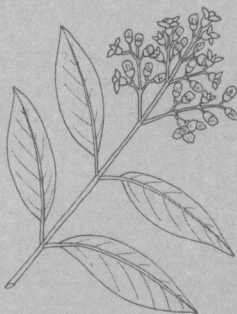

Sandalwood

Santalum album

MADE FROM:
Wood chips

APPEARANCE:
Thick, with pale yellow colouring

FRAGRANCE FAMILY:
Woody

KEY AROMAS:
Sweet, woody, soft, spicy

The scent of sandalwood has been present for millennia in rituals and religious practice, with the ancient Egyptians using it in incense and embalming. Sacred in Ayurvedic medicine, it is still widely used in important Hindu ceremonies and is revered for its purifying properties in traditional Eastern medicine.

This small, tropical tree has a distinctive aromatic timber which is widely used for furniture as well as in perfume, incense and for its essential oil, which is extracted from its wood chips by steam distillation.

Sandalwood's soft, warming scent is immensely comforting and eases mental tiredness as a result. Combined with its immune-boosting and skin-moisturizing qualities, it is a popular component of aromatherapy massage blends.

This oil with its spicy notes mixes well with other woody, spicy and resinous fragrances, such as cardamom, frankincense or myrtle, alongside slightly sharper citrus scents, such as lemon, grapefruit or neroli, which lift a blend.

Sandalwood uses

SUPPORTS RESPIRATORY SYSTEM
Helps defend against coughs, throat infections
and winter bugs.

BALANCES SKIN
Benefits dry or sun-damaged skin in particular.

CALMS THE MIND
Settles busy mental chatter; comforts
and reassures.

DETOXIFIES
Helps rid the body of toxins.

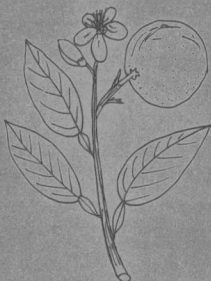

Sweet orange

Citrus sinensis

MADE FROM:
Peel of fruit

APPEARANCE:
Thin and yellow

FRAGRANCE FAMILY:
Citrus

KEY AROMAS:
Sweet, tangy, refreshing,
becoming softer as it evaporates

Oranges have been cultivated for more than 4,000 years and have long been popular for their medicinal as well as nutritional benefits, especially in ancient China where the peel was used to help with respiratory and digestive issues.

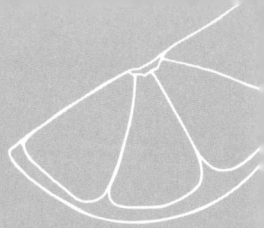

Sweet oranges are the fruit we most commonly eat as oranges, drink as juice and make into marmalade. In addition, its oil, which is extracted by expression from the peel of the fruit, is used widely as a flavouring in sweet foods and confectionery, and as a fragrance in toiletry products.

Sweet orange essential oil is used to soothe anxiety and gently elevate mood, as well as for its purifying qualities that aid the elimination of toxins from the body.

The tangy, orange aroma, lighter and a little less sharp than bitter orange, blends well with warm, woody scents, such as sandalwood and frankincense, alongside sweeter floral notes such as those from rose otto or Roman chamomile oil.

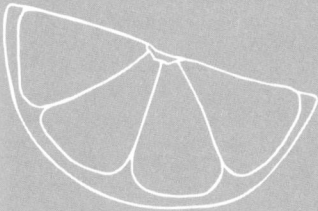

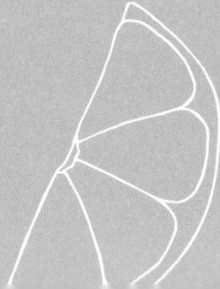

Orange uses

BOOSTS MOOD
Lifts the spirits and comforts the mind.

REJUVENATES SKIN
Revitalizes tired skin.

DETOXIFIES
Encourages the kidneys to remove toxins
from the system.

SOOTHES DIGESTION
Eases stomach aches and general
digestive discomfort.

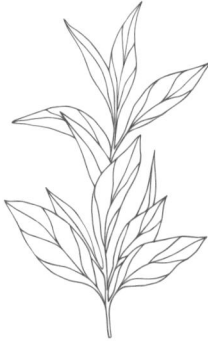

Tea tree

Melaleuca alternifolia

MADE FROM:
Leaves and twigs

APPEARANCE:
Very pale yellow

FRAGRANCE FAMILY:
Woody

KEY AROMAS:
Medicinal, green, fresh, cleansing

Native to Australia, the tea tree plant is a small tree or shrub with highly perfumed leaves and twigs from which the oil is extracted by steam distillation.

Long-used in indigenous medicine to combat colds and fevers, tea tree oil is now widely used and admired for its antiseptic, antibacterial and antimicrobial properties.

A popular natural ingredient in household cleaning products and insect repellents, tea tree's cleansing tones also work on the mind and emotions, refreshing the spirit and purging negativity.

The powerful and distinctive aroma of tea tree mixes best with other strong scents that can hold their own in a blend, such as patchouli, frankincense, lemon, myrrh and black pepper.

Tea tree uses

NOURISHES SCALP
Cleans, tones and balances the scalp if you add
a few drops to shampoo.

ACTS AS AN ANTIMICROBIAL CLEANSER
Helps fight throat and skin infections.

PROMOTES MENTAL HEALTH
Clears the mind, restores energy and
encourages optimism.

BOOSTS IMMUNITY
Supports body systems to repel viral infections.

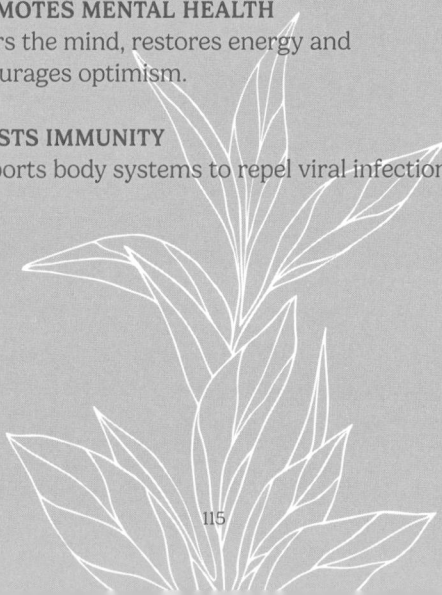

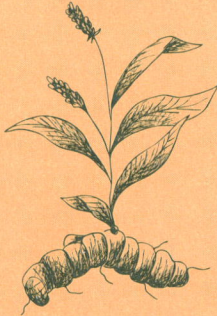

Turmeric

Curcuma longa

MADE FROM:
Roots

APPEARANCE:
Bright yellow oil

FRAGRANCE FAMILY:
Spicy

KEY AROMAS:
Warm, soft, spicy, a little earthy

Rich in vitamins, minerals and powerful antioxidants, turmeric is used to treat stomach disorders and skin issues in traditional Chinese medicine, while Ayurvedic medicine employs it to cleanse and detoxify the system.

Turmeric oil is extracted via steam distillation from the fleshy orange root of the turmeric plant, native to India and Southeast Asia.

Used as a cooking spice and in medicine for thousands of years, turmeric has antibacterial and antifungal properties and is known for its digestive and detoxifying benefits.

Gently warming, spicy and earthy, turmeric oil works well in blends with other warm aromas, such as frankincense, black pepper and coriander seed, when these are combined with a fresher scent with some sweetness, such as juniper berry, sweet orange or grapefruit

Turmeric uses

DETOXIFIES
Helps the body to purify itself and supports bowel health.

REPAIRS SKIN
Heals damaged skin, including issues such as ulcers and acne.

BOOSTS IMMUNITY
Helps maintain a healthy immune system and infection resistance.

AIDS DIGESTION
Tones digestion, helping with constipation, indigestion aches and cramps.

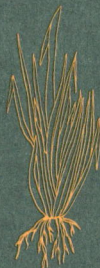

Vetiver

Vetiveria zizanoides

MADE FROM:
Roots

APPEARANCE:
Thick and dark brown

FRAGRANCE FAMILY:
Woody

KEY AROMAS:
Smoky, earthy, woody and deep
(lemon top note)

Extracted from the roots of this long, sharp-edged tropical grass via steam distillation, vetiver was harvested for oil in its native India as far back as the 12th century.

ESSENTIAL OILS

Vetiver oil is known for its calming and balancing effects on body and mind and is an excellent scent to use during a meditation practice. Its deep, sensual and relaxing aroma also speaks to its potency as an aphrodisiac.

Used widely in colognes and male grooming products, no doubt influenced by its earthy and heavy aroma, vetiver also has anti-inflammatory and antiseptic properties and soothes muscular pain.

The complex, powerful profile of vetiver oil blends well with similarly strong and heady scents, such as rose absolute, geranium, lavender, alongside spicier fragrances such as ginger and sandalwood.

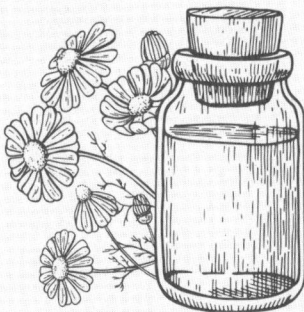

Vetiver uses

STABILIZES MOOD
Calms anxiety and emotional stress; grounding.

SOOTHES MUSCLES
Eases aches and pains, especially backache and muscle spasm.

TONES SKIN
Balances uneven or oily skin; restores tired-looking skin.

BOOSTS CIRCULATION
Supports the circulatory system and can ease stiffness.

BALANCES HORMONES
Soothes symptoms of PMS; evens out energy levels and combats menopausal tiredness.

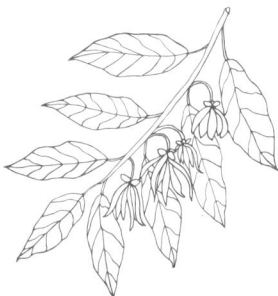

Ylang ylang

Cananga odorata

MADE FROM:
Yellow flowers

APPEARANCE:
Thin and colourless

FRAGRANCE FAMILY:
Floral

KEY AROMAS:
Sweet, floral, heady, with musky undertones

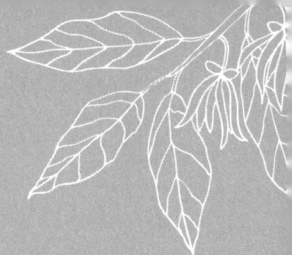

Ylang ylang is excellent for the hair and skin and was used by the Victorians in their Macassar Oil hair tonic.

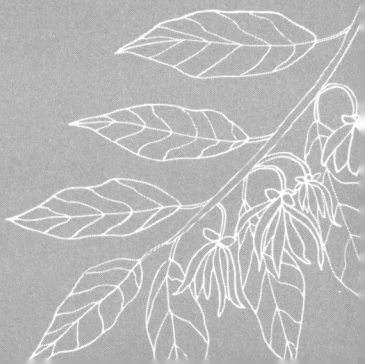

Native to Southeast Asia and Australasia, the evergreen climbing ylang ylang is sometimes called the "perfume tree", owing to the intoxicating sweet scent of its flowers.

It has large pink, mauve or yellow blooms. The yellow flowers are distilled to produce the oil because of their superior fragrance.

One of the most widely used plants in the perfume industry, ylang ylang's intensely floral scent lasts a long time on the skin and is prized for its soothing and aphrodisiacal properties.

A floral, musky oil with spicy undertones, ylang ylang blends well with other strong, sensual fragrances that won't be overpowered by it, such as patchouli, sandalwood, sweet orange, geranium, frankincense and may chang.

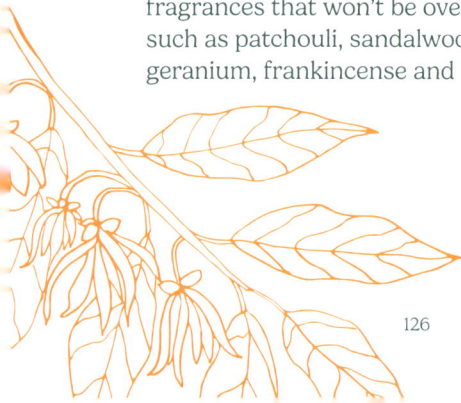

Ylang ylang uses

REVIVES SKIN AND HAIR
Conditions and tones the skin, hair and scalp.

ACTS AS AN APHRODISIAC
Relieves stress and thaws tense emotions.

CALMS THE MOOD
Eases irritability and comforts mind,
body and spirit.

SUPPORTS MENSTRUAL HEALTH
Balances out unpleasant symptoms,
especially PMS.

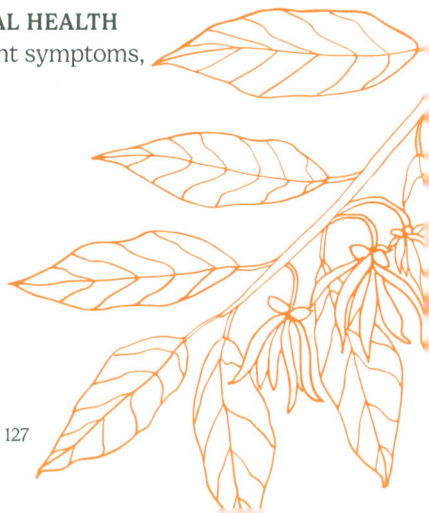

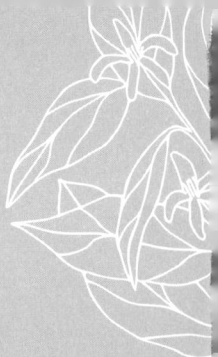

"Aromatherapy conveys
the concept of healing with
aromatic substances...
Because the oils work in a
different way from antibiotics,
they do not have the usual
side effects, and they tend to
stimulate the immune system
instead of depressing it."

Robert Tisserand,
Aromatherapy (1988)

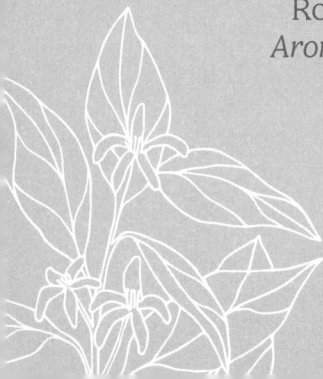